Things to Remember

There are many men with prostate cancer who have been in your shoes. Here are some things they would like you to know:

- There are treatment choices—be sure to know them all.

- Treatments and medical procedures keep getting better.

- Make the treatment choice that is right for you.

- Get the opinions of several different doctors, since some may suggest only the option they know best.

- Take the time you need to research your treatment choices before making a decision. There's often no need to rush.

- Your spouse or partner plays an important role in the treatment that you choose and will be affected by your choice. Try to be open and honest with each other about your concerns.

- Organizations and support groups can help you learn how others in your situation are coping with prostate cancer.

- It is possible to live a full life after prostate cancer.

Treatment Choices for Men With Early-Stage Prostate Cancer

3 Men . . .   3 Different Treatment Choices

"I talked it over with my wife and son. I chose **radiation therapy** because we thought it was the best choice for my situation."

"When my doctor said he would **follow me closely without treatment**, I thought he meant that I should give up. But after he explained my stage of cancer, it made sense to me. Now I know that I can decide to have treatment later."

"My wife and I looked at the benefits and risks of each treatment. After talking with several doctors who specialize in prostate cancer, we decided that **surgery** was the best choice for me."

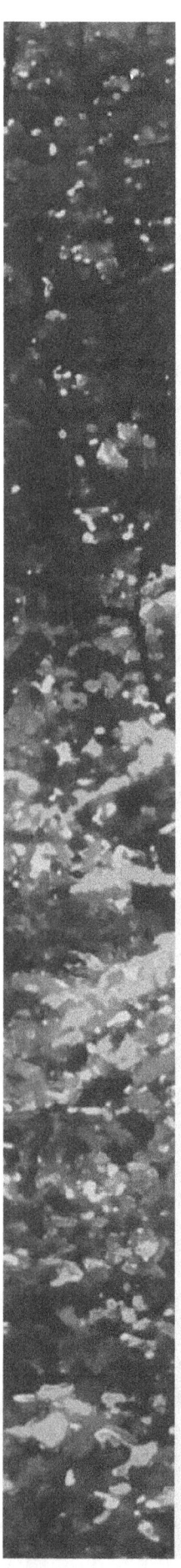
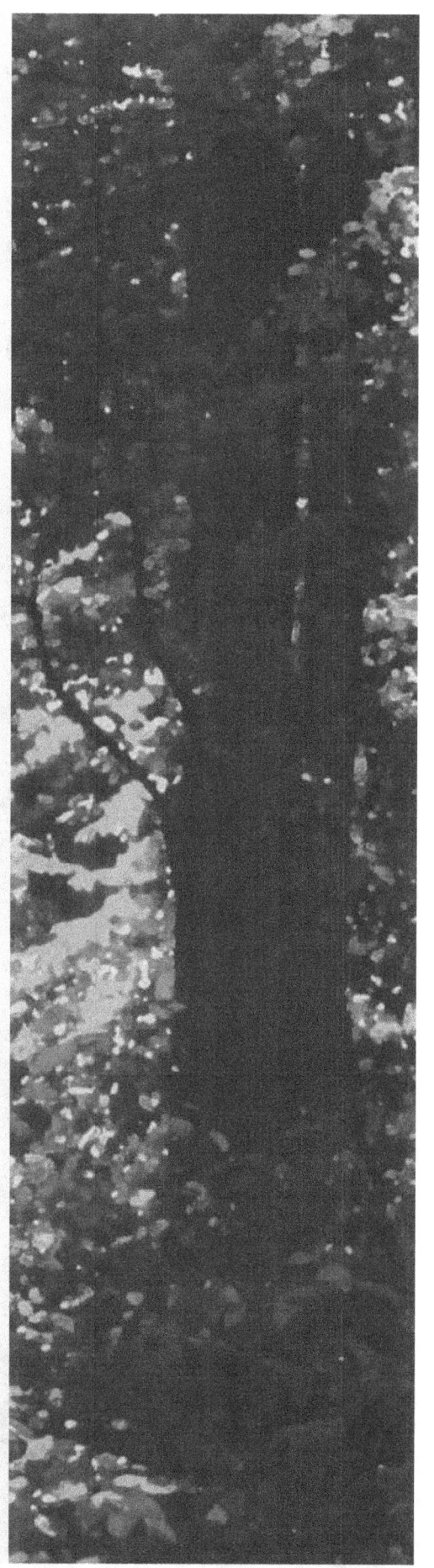

Table of Contents

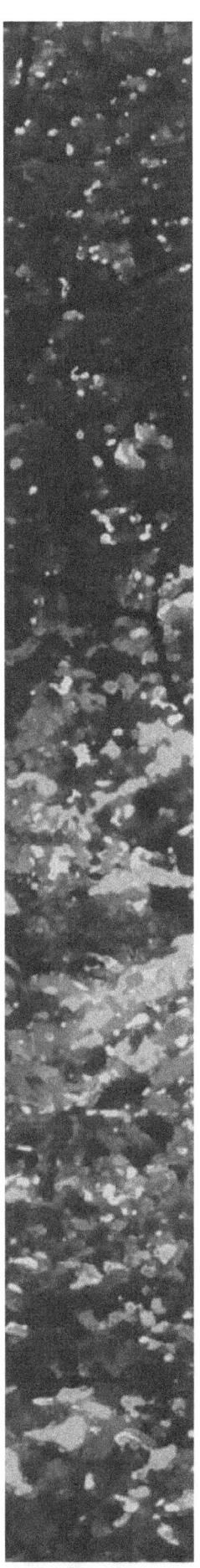

About This Booklet

As a man with early-stage **prostate cancer**, you will be able to choose which kind of treatment is best for you. And while it is good to have choices, this fact can make the decision hard to make. Yet, each choice has benefits (how treatment can help) and risks (problems treatment may cause).

Treatment often begins a few weeks to months after **diagnosis**. While you are waiting for treatment, you should meet with different doctors to learn about your treatment choices. Use this booklet to help you talk over treatment choices with your doctor before deciding which is best for you.

You will want to think about what is important to you. It's also a good idea to include your spouse or partner in your decision. After all, having prostate cancer and the treatment choice you make affect both of you.

Words that may be new to you appear in **bold** type. For a complete list of Words to Know, see pages 35 to 38.

This booklet is a starting point.

Its purpose is to help you learn about early-stage prostate cancer, different treatments, and the benefits and risks of each type of treatment. Most men will need more information than this booklet gives them to make a decision about treatment. For a list of groups that provide more information and support, please see the Ways to Learn More section on page 32. Also, see that section if you have prostate cancer that has spread beyond the prostate or that has returned after treatment.

What is the prostate?

The **prostate** is a gland that helps make semen. Semen is the milky fluid that carries sperm from the testicles through the penis during ejaculation. The prostate is part of the male reproductive system.

The prostate is about the size and shape of a walnut. It has sections, which are called lobes. The prostate lies low in the pelvis, below the bladder and in front of the rectum. The prostate surrounds part of the urethra, the tube that carries urine out of the bladder and through the penis.

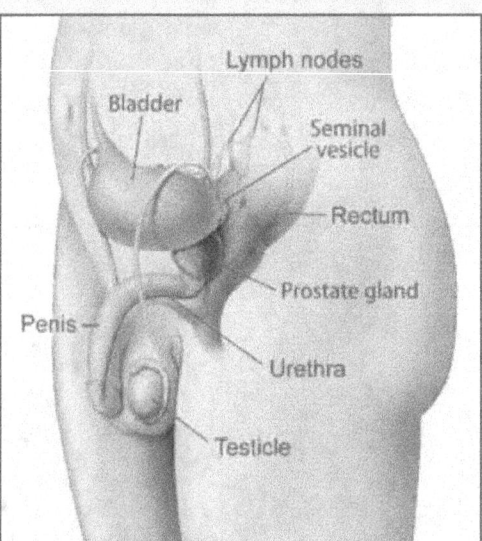

1-800-4-CANCER (1-800-422-6237)

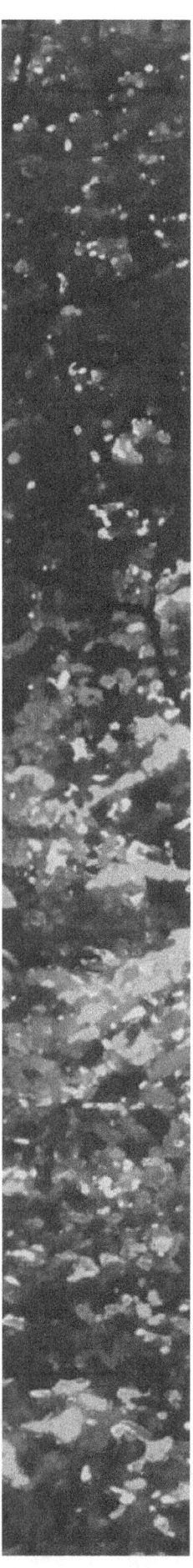

Facts About Prostate Cancer

Early-stage prostate cancer means that cancer cells are found only in your prostate. Compared with many other cancers, prostate cancer grows slowly. This means that it can take 10 to 30 years before a prostate tumor gets big enough to cause symptoms or for doctors to find it. Most men who have prostate cancer will die of something other than prostate cancer.

- Prostate cancer is most common in men age 65 and older, although younger men can be diagnosed with it as well.

- By age 80, more than half of all men have some cancer in their prostate.

- African American men tend to be diagnosed at younger ages and with faster-growing prostate cancer than men of other races.

Prostate cancer is most often found in early stages. When it is found early, there are a number of treatment choices available.

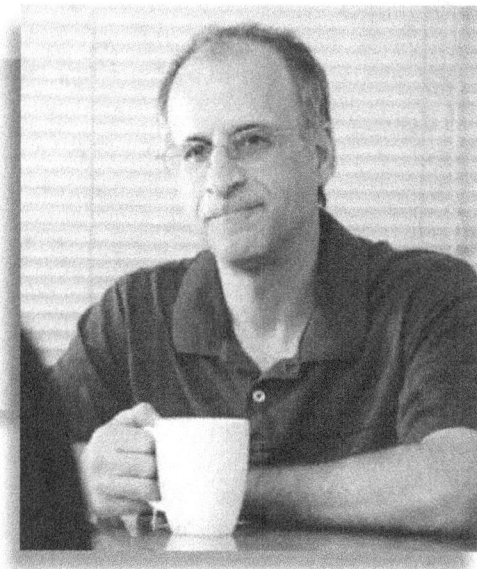

"Once I had enough information, I was better able to choose a treatment for me."
—Ken

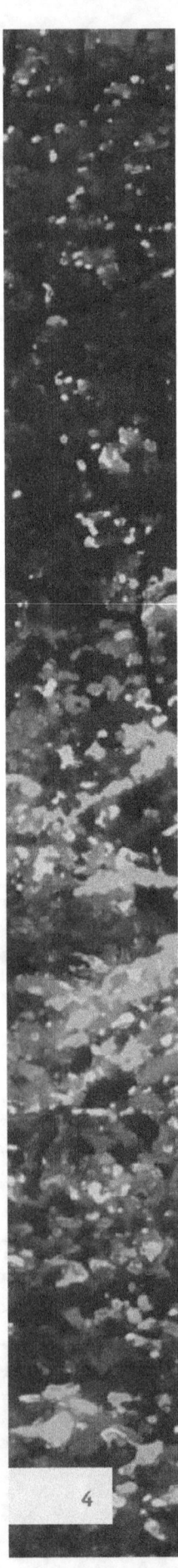

Thinking About Treatment Choices

Active surveillance, surgery, and **radiation therapy** are the **standard therapy** choices for men with early-stage prostate cancer (see Types of Treatment, starting on page 8). Each has benefits (how treatments can help) and risks (problems treatment may cause). There is seldom just one right treatment choice.

The choice of treatment depends on many factors:

■ **Your prostate cancer risk group.** Doctors use details about your cancer to place you into a low-, medium-, or high-risk group.

- **Low-risk** prostate cancer is not likely to grow or spread for many years.

- **Medium-risk** prostate cancer is not likely to grow or spread for a few years.

- **High-risk** prostate cancer may grow or spread within a few years.

Doctors define low-, medium-, and high-risk groups as follows:

	Low-Risk	Medium-Risk	High-Risk
PSA Level*	Less than 10 ng/ml**	10 to 20 ng/ml	More than 20 ng/ml
Gleason Score *(see page 6)*	6 or lower	7	8 or higher
Tumor Stage *(see page 7)*	T1 or T2a	T2b	T2c

*PSA stands for prostate-specific antigen (see page 6)

**ng/ml stands for nanograms per milliliter of blood

Reprinted with permission from:
1. Macmillan Publishers Ltd: Mazhar & Waxman. (2008) Nature Clinical Practice Urology 5: 486-493.
2. The American Medical Association: D'Amico, et al. (1998) JAMA 280 (11):969-974. Copyright © 1998 American Medical Association. All rights reserved.

1-800-4-CANCER (1-800-422-6237)

■ **Health problems other than prostate cancer.** Having heart problems, diabetes, or other illnesses may affect your treatment options.

■ **If you have already had surgery for an enlarged prostate.** If you have had prostate surgery, this may affect the treatment choices you have.

■ **Age.** The benefits and risks of different treatments may vary with age.

■ **Type of care available to you.** The skills and experience of specialists and types of treatment available in your area may vary. You will need to ask tough questions to make sure you receive the best possible care. See pages 30 and 31 for questions to ask.

■ **Thinking about what you value most.** Your unique experiences in life shape your feelings and thoughts about how to deal with prostate cancer. Keeping in mind what is important to you will help guide your decision.

Many men may ask their doctor, "What would you do, if you were me?" Try to remember, the doctor isn't you, and his or her personal values may be different from yours.

Here are some things to think about:

- How do you view the benefits and risks of the treatment choices that have been offered to you?

- Can you cope with knowing cancer is in your body?

- Would you rather have treatment to remove or shrink the cancer, knowing that there could be side effects?

- Do you know other men who have had prostate cancer? If so, their experiences may help you make your decision.

■ **Spouse or partner.** Even though the treatment choice is yours, involving your spouse, partner, or other loved ones can help you sort out what is most important to you and your family.

Medical Tests

By now you may have had many tests and exams to find out details about your cancer. As we discussed on pages 4 and 5, your doctor will take into account your general health, the results of your tests and exams, and the Gleason score of your cancer when talking with you about your treatment choices. What are these tests? What do their results mean?

- **Prostate-Specific Antigen (PSA) test.** PSA is a protein that is made by both normal prostate cells and prostate cancer cells. PSA is found in the blood and can be measured with a blood test. Because the amount of PSA in the blood often rises with prostate cancer, doctors may check your PSA level over time. If you have a score of 4ng/ml (which stands for nanograms per milliliter of blood) or higher, your doctor may want to do other tests, such as a prostate **biopsy**.

- **Gleason score of your cancer.** When you have a biopsy, samples are taken from many areas of your prostate. A doctor called a pathologist uses a microscope to check the samples for cancer. He or she assigns a Gleason score on a scale of 2 to 10 to your cancer. This score tells how different the prostate cancer tissue looks from normal prostate tissue and how likely it is that the cancer will grow or spread. Most men with early-stage prostate cancer have a Gleason score of 6 or 7.

- **Digital Rectal Exam (DRE).** In this exam, your doctor feels your prostate by inserting a gloved and lubricated finger into your rectum.

Stages of Early Prostate Cancer

The **clinical stage** of your cancer is important in choosing a treatment. The clinical stage tells how much the cancer may have grown within the prostate and whether it has spread to other tissues or organs. If you decide to have surgery, your prostate, nearby **lymph nodes**, and **seminal vesicles** will be removed and samples of them studied under a microscope. This exam gives the pathologist the information he or she needs to find out the **pathological stage** to your cancer.

Your doctor may do one or more of the following tests or exams to help figure out the stage of your cancer:

- DRE
- Prostate biopsy
- Bone scan
- MRI
- CT scan
- Biopsy of the lymph nodes in the pelvis
- Biopsy of the seminal vesicles

Tumor Stages

T1 means that the cancer is so small it can't be felt during a DRE. T1a and T1b cancer is most often found by accident, when men have surgery to relieve symptoms of BPH (which stands for **benign prostatic hyperplasia**).

T1c is most often found when a prostate biopsy is done because of a PSA test result that showed a high PSA blood level. This is the most commonly diagnosed stage of prostate cancer.

A stage of **T2** means that prostate cancer can be felt during a DRE, but is still only in the prostate. Your doctor may also assign a, b, or c to the stage, depending on the cancer's size and whether it is in 1 or more lobes of the prostate.

Stage
T1a

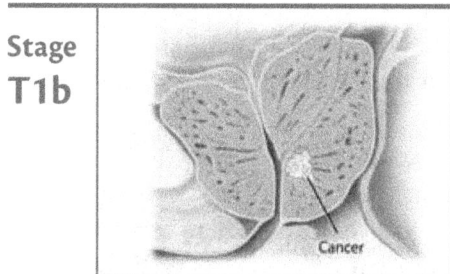

Stage
T1b

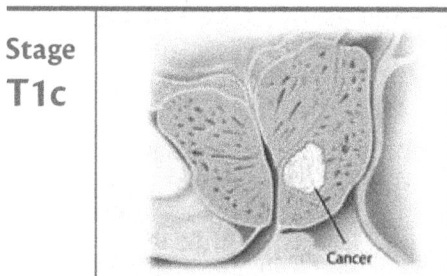

Stage
T1c

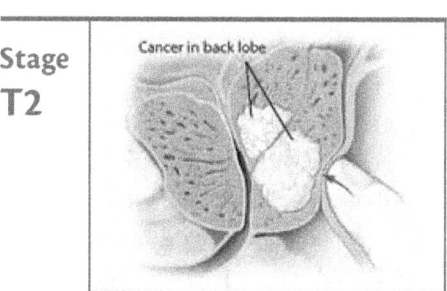

Stage
T2

Types of Treatment

Active Surveillance

Active surveillance is closely watching for any sign that the cancer may be growing or changing. You don't have to decide on a treatment right away. You will have frequent doctor visits and tests, such as DRE, PSA tests, and biopsies. If these tests show that your cancer is growing or changing in any way, your doctor will offer you radiation therapy or surgery to treat the cancer. You can also change your mind and decide to have treatment <u>at any time</u>.

Active surveillance can be used for men with early-stage prostate cancer because the cancer often grows so slowly that it may not cause problems during a man's lifetime. For some men, active surveillance may be a way to avoid the side effects and costs of treatment without shortening their life.

Surgery

Surgery is a treatment choice for men with early-stage prostate cancer who are in good health. Surgery to remove the prostate is called **prostatectomy**. There are different types of surgery for prostate cancer. They include:

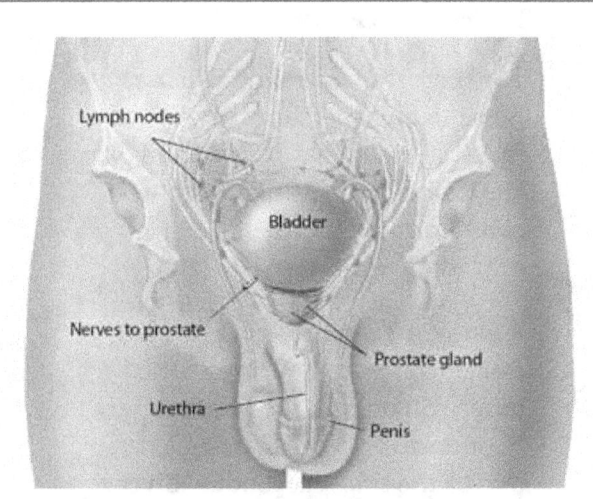

You may want to talk with your surgeon about techniques that may spare the nerves that control your bladder and erections.

- **Open prostatectomy.** Also called retropubic prostatectomy. In this surgery, your doctor removes the prostate through a single long cut made in your abdomen from a point below your navel to just above the pubic bone. He or she might also check nearby lymph nodes for cancer (see drawing below). This type of surgery can be used for **nerve-sparing surgery**. Nerve-sparing surgery lessens the chances that the nerves near your prostate will be harmed. These important nerves control erections and normal bladder function.

- **Laparoscopic surgery.** In this type of surgery, your doctor uses a laparoscope to see and remove the prostate. A laparoscope is a long slender tube with a light and camera on the end. This surgery is done through 4 to 6 small cuts in the navel and the abdomen, instead of a single long cut in the abdomen. The laparoscope is inserted through one of the cuts, and surgery tools are inserted through the others. A robot can be used to do this type of surgery. This type of surgery can also be used for nerve-sparing surgery.

- **Perineal prostatectomy.** In this type of surgery, your doctor removes the prostate through an incision between your **scrotum** and **anus**. With this method, the surgeon is not able to check the lymph nodes for cancer and nerve-sparing surgery is more difficult to do. This type of surgery is not used very often.

Radiation Therapy

This type of treatment uses high doses of radiation energy to treat cancer. Radiation therapy is a good choice for many men with early-stage prostate cancer. It is also the best treatment for older men or those who have other health problems. There are different types of radiation therapy:

- **External beam radiation.** In this type of radiation therapy, a machine aims radiation at your cancer. The machine moves around your body, sending radiation from many directions. Before you start treatment, your doctor will map out the exact location of your prostate. Then you will have treatment once a day, 5 days a week, for 6 to 9 weeks. Each treatment session usually lasts about 15 minutes.

  3-D conformal radiation therapy is a type of external beam radiation that is often used to treat prostate cancer. It allows doctors to carefully plan the shape of the radiation beam so it targets the cancer more precisely, while avoiding healthy tissues nearby.

- **Brachytherapy** is a type of internal radiation therapy in which a doctor places radioactive material inside the prostate. Brachytherapy is a choice for men with low-risk prostate cancer. There are two main types of brachytherapy used for prostate cancer, low-dose rate (also called LDR) and high-dose rate (also called HDR).

- **LDR brachytherapy.** In this type of brachytherapy, a doctor will place low-dose sources of radiation, or seed implants, throughout your prostate. Each seed implant is smaller than a grain of rice. The number of seeds will depend on the size of your prostate. The radiation will get weaker each day and run out in 2 to 10 months. Once the radiation is gone, the seeds will remain in your prostate, but they should not bother you. You will probably have the seeds implanted as an outpatient, without a hospital stay.

- **HDR brachytherapy.** Before treatment starts, a doctor will place tiny catheters (hollow tubes) throughout your prostate. For each treatment, the doctor will place 1 or more sources of high-dose radiation in the prostate through the catheters. Then, he or she will remove the radioactive material after a few minutes. The catheters will remain in place for the entire course of your treatment. But once you have received all of your treatments, the catheters will be removed. You will stay in the hospital or radiation clinic for the entire course of treatment.

External beam radiation therapy and brachytherapy can be used together.

For more information about external beam radiation and brachytherapy, see *Radiation Therapy and You: Support for People with Cancer,* a booklet from the National Cancer Institute. You can order a free copy at **www.cancer.gov/publications** or 1-800-4-CANCER (1-800-422-6237).

New Treatments

New treatments for prostate cancer are being studied in clinical trials, which are research studies with people. Clinical trials give people with any stage of cancer the chance to try a new treatment that is not yet available outside the trial. But until the clinical trials are complete, we do not know if the new treatments will be effective in the long-term.

> Until clinical trials are complete, we do not know if new treatments will be effective in the long-term.

Some treatments that researchers are studying for early-stage prostate cancer include:

- **Intensity-Modulated Radiation Therapy (IMRT).** IMRT is a type of external beam radiation. It uses computers to deliver radiation precisely to the cancer. It also reduces damage to the healthy tissue nearby, such as the rectum and bladder.

- **Proton beam therapy** is also a type of external beam radiation. It uses protons rather than x-rays. The use of protons may allow a very high dose of radiation to reach the prostate while reducing the amount of normal tissue that is affected.

- **Cryosurgery** (also called cryoablation or cryosurgical ablation) is a type of treatment that involves freezing the prostate to destroy cancer cells. In this type of treatment, the doctor delivers liquid nitrogen to the prostate through a special probe. The doctor inserts the probe into the prostate through an incision between the scrotum and anus. Sometimes, the doctor may also use needles to deliver liquid nitrogen to the prostate. He or she can insert the needles through the skin without making an incision.

 For more information about these treatments and other clinical trials, visit **www. cancer.gov/clinicaltrials** or call 1-800-4-CANCER (1-800-422-6237).

A Note About Hormone Therapy

Male sex hormones, such as **testosterone**, can help prostate cancer grow. **Hormone therapy** slows prostate cancer's growth by reducing the body's ability to make testosterone or by blocking testosterone's action in prostate cancer cells.

Hormone therapy can play a role in treating early-stage prostate cancer. For men with high-risk early-stage prostate cancer, it may be used along with radiation therapy. You can also receive it instead of surgery or radiation if:

- You are in your 70's or older or have other health problems
- Your cancer begins to change or grow while you are on active surveillance

Your doctor may suggest that you take hormone therapy for as little as 6 months or up to many years. Side effects may include loss of sex drive, **erectile dysfunction** (also called **ED**), hot flashes, and **osteoporosis**.

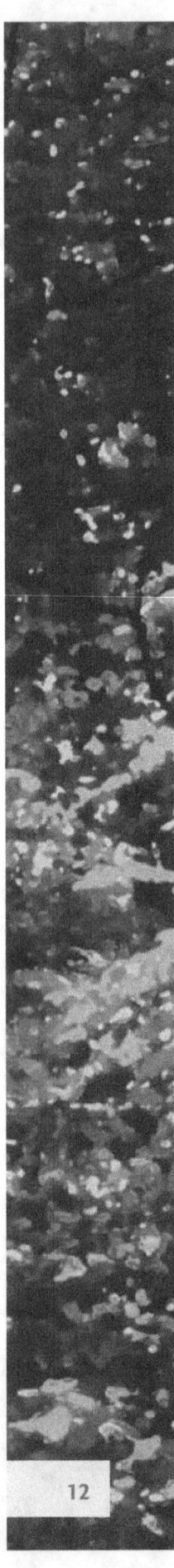

Comparing Your Treatment Choices

The charts on the following pages list 9 common questions and answers for the 3 treatment choices discussed in this booklet. As mentioned before, most men will need more information than found in this booklet to reach their decisions. You may use the questions in these charts as a guide for talking with your doctor or learning more about your choices.

Questions:	For answers see pages:
1. Which treatment is a good choice for me?	13
2. What can I expect during treatment?	14–15
3. What are the benefits of each treatment?	16
4. What are the side effects and other drawbacks of each treatment?	17–18
5. How will this treatment affect my sex life?	19
6. What can be done to help with side effects?	20–21
7. Will I have pain?	22
8. Will I need other treatments?	23
9. How long can I expect to live after I have this treatment?	24

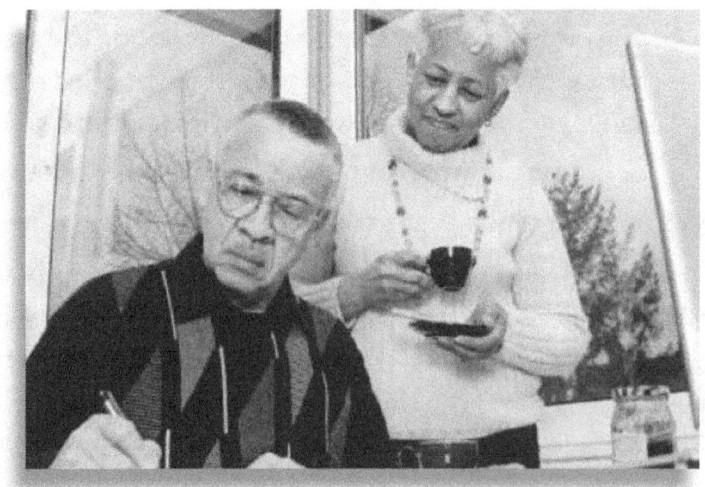

1-800-4-CANCER (1-800-422-6237)

1. Which treatment is a good choice for me?

Active Surveillance	■ If your cancer is:
	   • low-risk (see page 4)
	   • smaller or a slow-growing type of prostate cancer
	   • in the prostate only
	
	■ If you are in your 70s or older, or have serious medical problems.
	
	■ If you are able to accept the fact that the cancer will remain in your body.
	
	■ If you can be careful about always going to your check-ups.

Surgery	■ If you are younger than 70 and in good health. ■ If you want the cancer to be removed. ■ If you are able to accept that you might have serious side effects. ■ If you are able to accept that you may still need radiation therapy after your surgery.
Radiation Therapy	■ If you are a man of any age with early-stage prostate cancer. ■ If you have serious health problems that do not allow you to have surgery. ■ If you are able to go for treatment 5 days a week for up to 9 weeks. ■ If you have high-risk cancer (see page 4) that is less likely to be cured by surgery alone.

2. What can I expect during treatment?

Active Surveillance	■ You will not start treatment right away. ■ You will have frequent visits to the doctor. ■ You and your doctor will watch for signs that the cancer may be changing or growing. You will have: • Frequent DRE and PSA tests, usually every 3 months • Biopsies every 1 to 3 years
Surgery	■ Surgery takes about 2 to 4 hours. ■ Most patients stay in the hospital for 2 to 4 days. ■ The doctor will remove the entire prostate, the seminal vesicles, and a small part of the bladder.
Radiation Therapy	■ **External Beam Radiation** • Your doctor will figure out the dose of the radiation to the cancer with the least damage to the normal tissue nearby. • You will lie on a table while a large machine aims radiation at your cancer. • You will have no pain or discomfort. • You will have treatment once a day, 5 days a week, for up to 9 weeks. ■ **Brachytherapy** **LDR brachytherapy** • Your doctor will insert radioactive seeds (each smaller than a grain of rice) into the prostate or surrounding area. He or she will implant the seeds using hollow needles inserted through the space between the scrotum and the anus. *continued on next page*

1-800-4-CANCER (1-800-422-6237)

Radiation Therapy *continued*

- You will be numbed below the waist or put to sleep.
- It takes an hour or so for the doctor to implant the seeds.
- You will spend a total of 5 to 6 hours in the hospital and should not need to spend the night.
- The seeds will stay in your body even after the radiation is gone.
- While the seeds are giving off radiation you should avoid being near children or pregnant women.

HDR brachytherapy

- A doctor will insert tiny catheters into the prostate or surrounding area.
- The doctor will deliver a radioactive source to the prostate through the catheter and remove it after a short time.
- Most people have 3 treatments over 24 hours.
- You will remain in the hospital until you have finished all of your treatments.
- Once you have finished your treatments, the catheters will be removed.

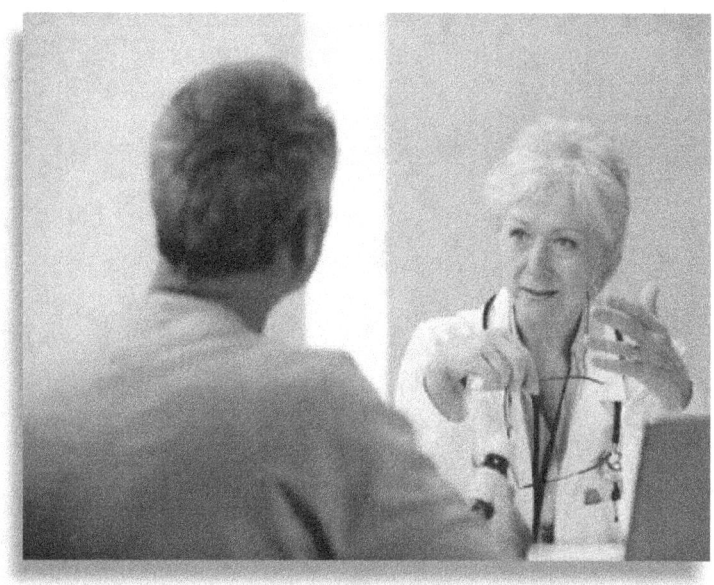

3. What are the benefits of each treatment?

Active Surveillance	▪ You will have no side effects. ▪ Your doctor will follow you closely and you will have regular check-ups. ▪ You can decide to begin treatment at any time.
Surgery	▪ The prostate cancer is removed by removing as much of the prostate as possible.
Radiation Therapy	▪ **External Beam Radiation** • You will not need to spend the night in the hospital. • You will not need to be numbed below the waist or put to sleep. • You may have fewer problems with urination than if you have surgery. ▪ **Brachytherapy** • For LDR brachytherapy, you will not need to spend the night in the hospital. • It can be easier on your body than surgery. • There will likely be less damage to the rectum and nearby tissue than with external beam radiation.

4. What are the side effects and other drawbacks of each treatment?

Active Surveillance	■ You may have feelings of worry and anxiety about living with cancer and putting off treatment. ■ The cancer needs to be followed closely. ■ You will have frequent tests, such as blood tests and biopsies. ■ The cancer could spread and become harder to treat.
Surgery	■ There are risks with any major surgery, such as pain, bleeding, infection, heart problems, or death. ■ It takes longer to recover than it does with radiation therapy. ■ For 1 to 2 weeks after surgery, you will need to use a catheter (a hollow tube) to pass your urine. ■ You may have problems with **incontinence**, which means you are not able to control the flow of urine. Managing this problem often means wearing pads, such as Depend® pads, to catch urine. The most common type of incontinence is passing a small amount of urine from the stress of coughing, laughing, or sneezing. A small number of men may have more serious incontinence that can last the rest of their life. ■ Most men will have trouble getting an erection right after surgery, a problem called impotence, erectile dysfunction, or ED. This may improve over 1 to 2 years. Erectile dysfunction may occur if the cancer is close to the nerves that control erections. If these nerves are damaged or removed during surgery, there is a strong chance that you will have problems with erectile dysfunction after surgery. Other factors that affect erectile dysfunction are your age, medicines you take, your hormone levels, other health problems, and how strong your erections were before surgery.

continued on next page

4. What are the side effects and other drawbacks of each treatment option? *continued*

Radiation Therapy	■ **External Beam Radiation**
	
	During Treatment
	• Fatigue (being very tired) toward the end of your course of treatment
	• More frequent and softer bowel movements
	• Urinary problems, such as needing to go more urgently and more often, especially at night
	• Irritation or bleeding from your rectum
	
	After Treatment
	• You may develop erectile dysfunction within 5 years of treatment. Half of the men who have radiation therapy will develop problems with erectile dysfunction that are like those seen with surgery.
	• You may develop bowel problems, such as diarrhea, trouble controlling bowel movements, and rectal bleeding.
	• You may feel discomfort in the bladder or rectal area.
	• Your PSA may go up for a short time.
	
	■ **Brachytherapy**
	
	During Treatment
	• More frequent and urgent need to pass urine
	• More discomfort when passing urine
	• Bowel problems, such as diarrhea, trouble controlling bowel movements, and rectal bleeding
	
	After Treatment
	• You may develop problems with:
	  – Emptying your bladder
	  – Dribbling of urine
	  – Erectile dysfunction, similar to that found with surgery

5. How will this treatment affect my sex life?

Active Surveillance	■ It should not affect your sex life.
Surgery	■ Surgery to remove the prostate can cause erectile dysfunction. Talk with your doctor about whether nerve-sparing surgery can be used to limit damage to the nerves that control erections. Medications and devices can help many men with erectile dysfunction (see page 20). ■ After your prostate is removed, your orgasm may be "dry," which means that you will make little, if any, semen. If you want to have children in the future, you will need to bank your sperm before surgery. Banking your sperm means freezing it for future use. See Ways to Learn More on page 32 for more information.
Radiation Therapy	■ You are just as likely to develop problems with erectile dysfunction as you are with surgery. But, these problems will develop 3 to 5 years after treatment, rather than right after. Your age and health can also affect problems you might have with erectile dysfunction.

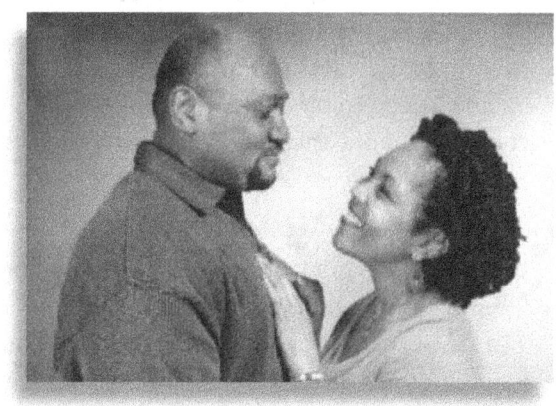

6. What can be done to help with side effects?

Active Surveillance	■ You will have no side effects

Surgery	■ **For erectile dysfunction**
	• There are medicines you can take by mouth that can increase blood flow to the penis, leading to an erection. They work best for men who have had nerve-sparing surgery. These medicines include:
	  – Sildenafil (Viagra®)
	  – Vardenafil (Levitra®)
	  – Tadalafil (Cialis®)
	• There are also medicines you can give yourself with a shot into the penis. Once you give yourself the shot, it will take about 5 minutes to start working and the effect will last for 20 to 90 minutes.
	• If medicine you take by mouth or shots do not help you, you should talk with your doctor about other choices. Other choices that may lead to an erection include:
	  – **Medicated urethral system for erection**, also called **MUSE**, in which you insert a small pellet into your urethra using an applicator.
	  – Vacuum erection devices, which use a vacuum tube connected to a pump to help produce an erection. The pump helps blood flow to the penis.
	  – Penile implants, which are devices that are placed inside the penis through surgery. Implants can be firm rods or devices that inflate.
	• You may need to try different treatments or combination of treatments in order to find something that works for you.
	
	■ **For incontinence**
	• Lack of bladder control may be severe for about 6 to 12 weeks after surgery. During this time, you will need to wear an absorbent pad, such as a Depend® pad.
	• Emptying your bladder often may help to control leaks. Other choices for managing incontinence include collection devices, **biofeedback**, and surgery.
	
	continued on next page

Surgery *continued*	• Collection devices consist of a pouch or condom-like device that is securely placed around the penis. A drainage tube is attached at the tip of the device to remove urine. The drainage tube empties into a storage bag, which can be emptied directly into a toilet.
Radiation Therapy	■ **Urinary problems** • Talk with your doctor or nurse if you have urinary problems. He or she may refer you to a physical therapist who will assess your problem. The therapist can give you exercises to improve bladder control. • Your doctor may prescribe medicines that can help you urinate, reduce burning or pain, and ease bladder spasms. ■ **For diarrhea** • Drink plenty of clear liquids. After you have a bowel movement, clean yourself with moist wipes, instead of toilet paper. • Try eating smaller meals and snacks, instead of 3 large meals. Also, eat foods that are easy on the stomach. Avoid fried, greasy, and spicy foods, and those that are high in fiber, such as raw fruits and vegetables.

For more information about dealing with problems caused by radiation therapy, see *Radiation Therapy and You: Support for People with Cancer,* a booklet from the National Cancer Institute. You can order a free copy at **www.cancer.gov/publications** or 1-800-4-CANCER (1-800-422-6237).

7. Will I have pain?

Active Surveillance	■ You will have frequent tests, such as blood tests and biopsies, which may cause some discomfort.
Surgery	■ Some men have little pain after surgery, but others need pain relief. There are medicines that can help control pain after surgery. Be sure to tell your doctor or nurse if you need help.
Radiation Therapy	■ **External beam radiation therapy** • External beam radiation therapy itself does not cause pain, but over time it can cause side effects that cause discomfort in the bladder or rectal area. If you do have pain, be sure to tell your doctor or nurse. ■ **Brachytherapy** • You might feel mild pain where the seeds were implanted. • You might feel burning or pain when you pass urine.

Medicines can help with pain or discomfort. Be sure to talk with your doctor or nurse about your pain.

For more information about pain and how to manage it, see *Pain Control: Support for People with Cancer,* a booklet from the National Cancer Institute. You can order a free copy at **www.cancer.gov/publications** or 1-800-4-CANCER (1-800-422-6237).

8. Will I need other treatments?

Active Surveillance	▪ If tests show that your cancer is growing or changing, you may need surgery or radiation therapy. If you do not want to go through surgery or radiation therapy, are older or have other health problems, hormone therapy may be a good choice for you.
Surgery	▪ Your doctor might suggest you have radiation therapy after you have had surgery. ▪ Within 5 years of surgery, the blood level of PSA will start to go up again in about 1 out of 3 men. If your PSA level begins to rise, it may be a sign that your cancer has come back. If that happens, your treatment choices may include: • Active surveillance • Hormone therapy • Radiation therapy, especially if your PSA level is less than 1 ng/ml
Radiation Therapy	▪ If you have high-risk cancer, hormone therapy may be used to shrink the prostate before radiation therapy. You might also take it for many years after radiation therapy. ▪ Within 5 years of radiation therapy, the blood level of PSA will start to go up again in about 1 out of 3 men. If your PSA level begins to rise, your treatment choices will most likely include active surveillance or hormone therapy. Less often, your doctor may suggest surgery or cryotherapy.

For more information about treatment choices or clinical trials for prostate cancer, visit NCI's Web site at **www.cancer.gov/cancertopics/types/prostate** or call the National Cancer Institute's Cancer Information Service toll-free at 1-800-4-CANCER (1-800-422-6237).

9. How long can I expect to live after I have this treatment?

Active Surveillance, Surgery, and Radiation Therapy

■ Most men with early-stage prostate cancer can expect to have many healthy years ahead of them. The average age for men to learn they have early-stage prostate cancer is 65 years. For all 3 treatments:
- Nearly all men will still be alive 5 years after treatment.
- 86% of men will still be alive 10 years after treatment.
- 56% of men will still be alive 15 years after treatment.

■ Even if the cancer comes back, there are many treatments that can help.

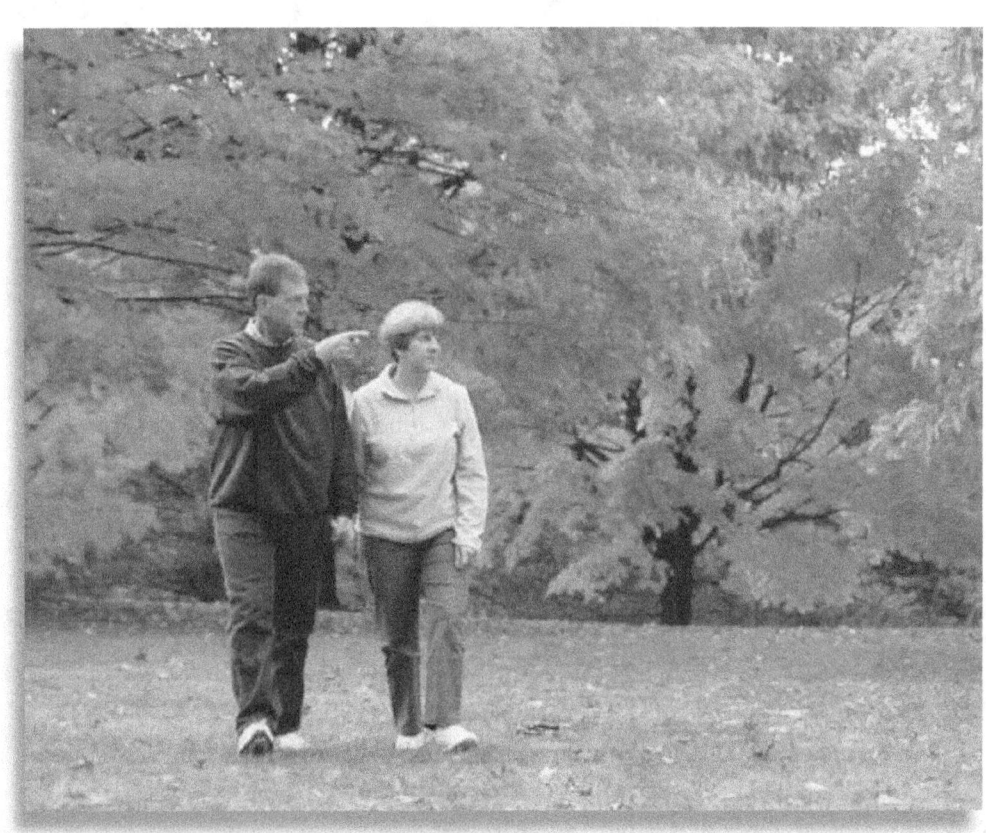

1-800-4-CANCER (1-800-422-6237)

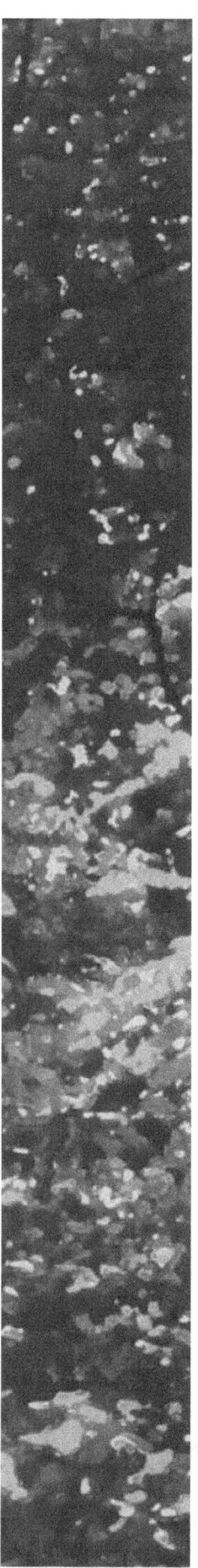

Choosing Your Treatment

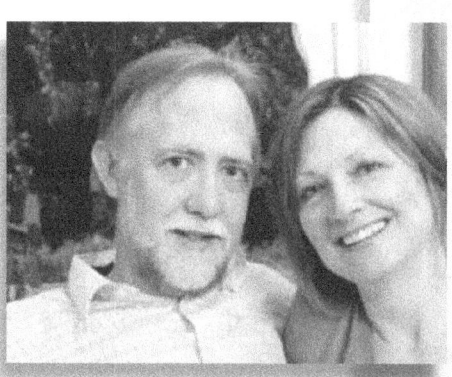

I looked at all my choices and was comfortable with the decision I made. I took my time because I didn't want to second-guess myself once it was all over. —Lawrence

Most prostate cancers found in the early stages grow slowly. This means that you usually do not have to rush to make a treatment choice. Often, you have many weeks to many months from the time you first learn you have prostate cancer until you have to make a choice.

Many men use this time to find out more about the different types of prostate cancer treatment. Be sure to find all of the information you need to answer your questions and be comfortable with your decision.

It may be helpful to use this extra time to attend a prostate cancer support group to talk with other men who have faced the same decision-making process. Think about calling the National Cancer Institute's toll-free number to request contact information for prostate cancer organizations. See page 32 for ways to reach them.

Research shows that men feel better about their treatment choice when they take part in making their own treatment decision. Making this decision can be hard to do. The following are some ideas that may help.

Be prepared when you talk with your doctor.

■ **Ask Questions.** Ask your doctor or nurse questions that you are thinking about, even if you are not comfortable asking them. These questions can be about topics that are new to you or side effects that concern you. Write your questions down and bring them to your doctor visit. (See pages 30 and 31 for ideas of questions to ask.)

- **Know your health history.** Your doctor or nurse will want to know about your health history. This history includes your family history, whether you have already had prostate surgery, and whether you have any other illness, such as diabetes or heart problems.

- **Talk about your treatment choices.** It's important to ask your doctors about all the treatment choices that are open to you. This includes benefits (how each treatment can help) and long- and short-term side effects.

- **Take part in making a choice.** Men who take an active part in their treatment tend to feel better about their treatment than men who let others decide for them. Let your doctor know how active you want to be in making this choice.

- **Think about what is important to you.** Keep in mind what's important to you and what worries you. This is also a good time for you and your spouse or partner to have an open, honest discussion with each other about your treatment choices and their possible side effects.

- **Ask a family member or trusted friend or caregiver to come to doctor visits with you.** This person can help listen, ask questions, take notes, and talk with you about what your doctor or nurse said.

- **Get a copy of your pathology report.** Ask your doctor for a copy of this report and bring a copy with you when you see new doctors. Your pathology report includes the results of tests that describe details about your cancer. If you are seeing a new doctor, it's important to bring all the information he or she requests to your visit.

When I was first faced with this decision, I was so confused I wanted to put myself in the hands of an expert. But, I knew it was a decision I had to make. Getting more than one opinion helped me make an informed choice. —Paul

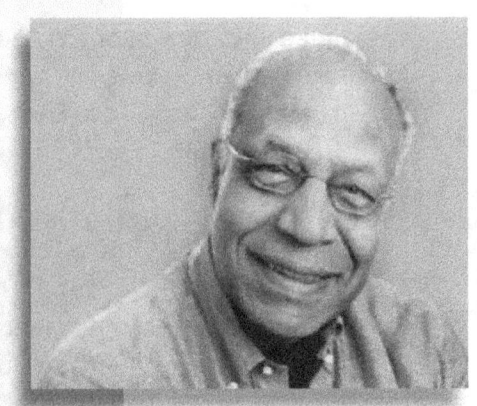

1-800-4-CANCER (1-800-422-6237)

■ **Get a 2nd or even 3rd opinion.** Seeking other opinions means talking about prostate cancer treatment with other doctors. You may want to talk with other prostate cancer specialists, such as those listed at the bottom of this page.

Getting 2nd and 3rd opinions can be confusing because you may get different advice. Because of this, many men find it helpful to see a medical oncologist for a general view of prostate cancer treatment choices. Talking with other doctors can give you ideas to think about or help you feel better about the choice you are making. Most insurance companies pay for 2nd opinions. Some companies even require them. It is better to get a 2nd opinion than to worry that you made the wrong choice.

Many cancer centers allow men to meet with a urologist, radiation oncologist, medical oncologist, and pathologist in one visit. Check to see if your treatment center provides this type of care.

Types of Doctors

Here is a list of types of doctors who treat prostate cancer:

■ **Medical oncologist.** A doctor who specializes in diagnosing and treating cancer using chemotherapy, hormone therapy, and biological therapy. This doctor is often the main health care provider for people with cancer. He or she can also treat side effects and may coordinate treatment given by other specialists.

■ **Pathologist.** A doctor who finds diseases by studying cells and tissue under a microscope. Although you won't meet with this doctor, he or she writes up a pathology report, which contains the information about your cancer from your biopsy or prostate surgery.

■ **Radiation oncologist.** A doctor who treats cancer with radiation.

■ **Urologic oncologist.** A doctor who treats cancers of the urinary system.

■ **Urologist.** A doctor who treats diseases of the urinary system and male sex organs.

Learning as Much as You Want to Know

Many men with prostate cancer find that it helps to learn a lot about their cancer and its treatment. Doing so can help you feel more in control and at ease with the treatment you choose.

You can learn more by reading books and articles, searching the internet, or calling organizations that focus on prostate cancer. But keep in mind that too much information can be overwhelming as you are adjusting to your diagnosis. Instead, learn as much as you want to know when you are ready. Later, you can always find out more. Let your doctor or nurse know what else you need to know to be comfortable reaching a decision.

Some men want to read books and articles about the current research on prostate cancer treatment choices. Others prefer to meet with men in support groups who have had prostate cancer to learn how they made their treatment choices. Some men may not want to talk or think about it, at first. But later, they are they ready for more information. All of these approaches are natural ways to cope with a diagnosis of prostate cancer.

 *To learn more* about finding information on the internet see the fact sheet "How to Evaluate Health Information on the Internet" at **http://www.cancer.gov/cancertopics/factsheet/Information/internet**. Also see Ways to Learn More on page 32.

Thinking About Your Feelings and Values

It's normal to have many feelings at this time. You may have many strong feelings at once. You may feel overwhelmed or angry. Your spouse or partner will also feel a range of feelings, but not have the same ones at the same time as you do.

Finding out you have cancer can bring up fears of the cancer getting worse or of dying. You may also worry about changes to your body or being intimate with your spouse or partner. Many men describe a feeling of loss—loss of the life they had before cancer, loss of energy levels, or the physical loss of the prostate. These feelings are a normal part of the coping process.

Your spouse or partner may be worried about losing you, changes to your lives, and how to best give you the support you need. At first, your loved one may want to talk about it more than you do. If you find that you need time to adjust and sort out your feelings and values, let your spouse or partner and family know your needs. Chances are that they are also trying to cope with the news and may not know how best to help you. If you are holding your worries and feelings inside for too long and your silence is hurting you or your family, ask your doctor, counselor, or religious leader for suggestions about getting help.

Reaching a decision about how you want to treat your prostate cancer is very personal—it is a balance of what is important to you, what you value the most, what types of treatment choices are available to you, and what the benefits and risks are.

Talking With Others

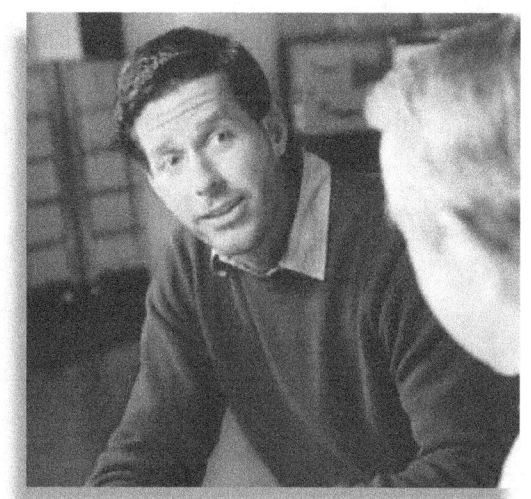

Along with talking with their doctors and spouse or partner, many men find it helpful to talk with others, such as:

■ **Family.** This includes your relatives and close friends who care about you. They can support your treatment choice.

■ **Men who have faced prostate cancer.** There is a lot to learn from other men who have faced these same prostate cancer treatment decisions. You may want to join a support group or meet with others to talk about the choices they made and what life is like now that treatment is over. Remember that while your stage of prostate cancer may be the same as someone else's, your life and desires may be very different.

■ **Others who can help.** You may have other people in your life who can help. This may be a neighbor, counselor, social worker, or religious leader you like and trust.

Asking Questions

You may find it helpful to ask the following questions:

■ What is the clinical stage and Gleason score of my cancer? _____

■ Is my cancer low-, medium-, or high-risk?

    ☐ Low-risk

    ☐ Medium-risk

    ☐ High-risk

■ What treatment do you recommend?

    ☐ Active surveillance

    ☐ Surgery (What type of surgery? Can the nerves be spared? How often do you do this procedure?)

    _____

    _____

    ☐ Radiation (What type of radiation? What can be done to reduce side effects?)

    _____

    _____

    ☐ Other

    _____

    _____

■ What are the short- and long-term side effects of this treatment?

_____

_____

■ What are my chances of:

    ☐ Becoming incontinent?_____

    ☐ Developing ED? _____

    ☐ Having other bladder or bowel problems?_____

1-800-4-CANCER (1-800-422-6237)

■ What are the chances of the cancer coming back if I have this treatment?

_____

_____

_____

■ What are my chances of survival?

_____

_____

_____

■ May I have a copy of my pathology report? _____

■ If I want to have another pathologist look at my prostate biopsy results, how do I get the slides?

_____

_____

_____

Making a Choice

"Prostate cancer gives you the opportunity to make a deliberate, considered choice. In the majority of cases, the disease is very slow growing and is never a medical emergency. With prostate cancer, you have ample time to assess the situation, evaluate your particular needs and resources, and devise the most sensible, strategic plan of action. Doctors can and should help you to understand your medical situation, but only you can decide what trade-offs you can tolerate, what level of risk you find acceptable, and which potential sacrifices you're willing to make."

—Dr. Peter Scardino, Chairman of the Department of Urology, Memorial Sloan Kettering Cancer Center

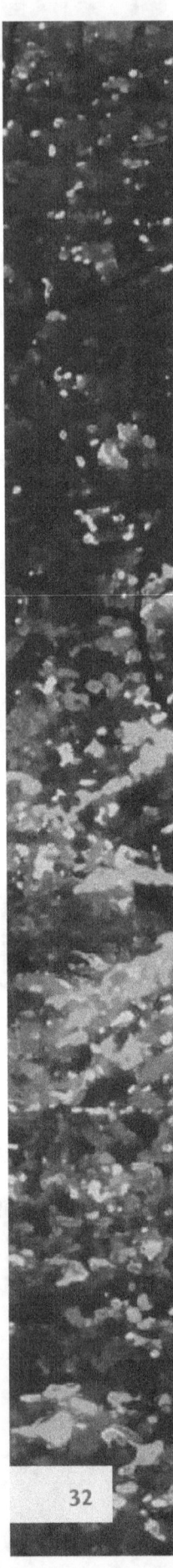

Ways to Learn More

National Cancer Institute (NCI)

You can find out more from these free NCI services:

Call: 1-800-4-CANCER (1-800-422-6237)

Visit: www.cancer.gov

Chat: www.cancer.gov/livehelp

Email: cancergovstaff@mail.nih.gov

Free booklets that are available include:

- *What You Need To Know About Prostate Cancer*
- *Radiation Therapy and You: Support for People With Cancer*
- *Pain Control: Support for People With Cancer*
- *When Someone You Love Is Being Treated for Cancer: Support for Caregivers*

Other Federal Resources

Medicare

Call: 1-800-MEDICARE (1-800-633-4227)

Visit: www.medicare.gov

National Kidney and Urologic Diseases Information Clearinghouse

Call: 1-800-891-5390

Visit: www.kidney.niddk.nih.gov

Other Organizations

American Cancer Society Man-to-Man Program

This support group of the American Cancer Society offers advice on coping with illness and the side effects of treatment, along with newsletter archives and a directory of prostate cancer publications.

Call: 1-800-ACS-2345 (1-800-227-2345)

Visit: www.cancer.org

American Urological Association Foundation

The AUA Foundation supports research; provides education to patients, the general public, and health professionals; and offers patient support services for those who have or may be at risk for a urologic disease or disorder. The Foundation provides information on urologic diseases and dysfunctions, including prostate cancer treatment choices, bladder health, and sexual function. It also offers prostate cancer support groups (Prostate Cancer Network). Some Spanish language publications are available.

Call: 1-800-828-7866

Visit: www.urologyhealth.org

The Cancer Support Community

Dedicated to providing support, education, and hope to people affected by cancer.

Call: 1-888-793-9355

Visit: www.cancersupportcommunity.org

Email: help@cancersupportcommunity.org

CancerCare

CancerCare is a national nonprofit agency that offers free support, information, financial assistance, and practical help to people with cancer and their loved ones. Services are provided by oncology (cancer) social workers and are available in person, over the telephone, and through the agency's Web site. A section of the CancerCare Web site and some publications are available in Spanish, and staff can respond to calls and e-mail in Spanish.

Call: 1-800-813-HOPE (1-800-813-4673)

Visit: www.cancercare.org

Fertile Hope

Fertile Hope is a national organization that provides reproductive information, support, and hope to cancer patients whose medical treatments present the risk of infertility. The organization offers fertility preservation financial assistance choices for patients.

Call: 1-866-965-7205

Visit: www.fertilehope.org

Prostate Cancer Foundation

The Prostate Cancer Foundation is a nonprofit organization that provides funding for research projects to improve methods of diagnosing and treating prostate cancer. It also offers printed resources for prostate cancer survivors and their families. The mission of the Prostate Cancer Foundation is to find better treatments and a cure for prostate cancer.

Call: 1-800-757-CURE (1-800-757-2873)

Visit: www.prostatecancerfoundation.org

Us TOO International

Us TOO International Prostate Cancer Education and Support Network is a non-profit education and support group organization with more than 325 chapters throughout the world. It provides men and their families with fellowship, peer counseling, and timely, personalized, unbiased, and reliable information about prostate cancer, enabling informed choices about detection, treatment choices, and quality of life after treatment.

Call: 1-800-80-USTOO (1-800-808-7866)

Visit: www.ustoo.org

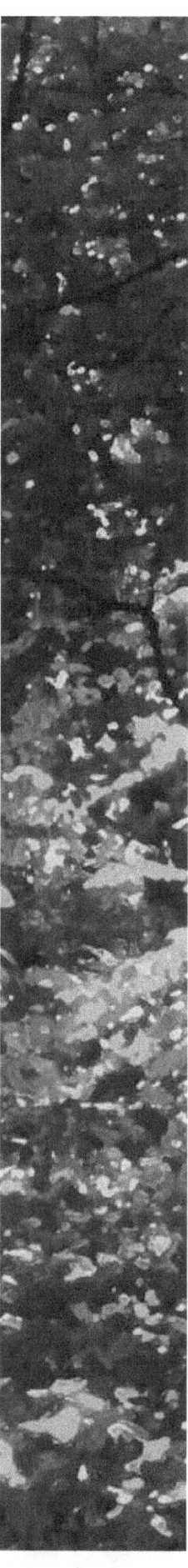

Words to Know

3-D conformal radiation therapy (3-D kun-FOR-mul RAY-dee-AY-shun THAYR-uh-pee): A procedure that uses a computer to create a three-dimensional picture of the tumor. This allows doctors to give the highest possible dose of radiation to the tumor, while sparing the normal tissue as much as possible. Also called 3-dimensional radiation therapy.

Active surveillance (AK-tiv ser-VAY-lents): Closely watching a patient's condition but not giving treatment unless there are changes in test results.

Anus (AY-nus): The opening of the rectum to the outside of the body.

Benign prostatic hyperplasia (beh-NINE prah-STA-tik HY-per-PLAY-zhuh): A benign (not cancer) condition in which an overgrowth of prostate tissue pushes against the urethra and the bladder, blocking the flow of urine. Also called BPH.

Biofeedback: A method of learning to voluntarily control certain body functions such as heartbeat, blood pressure, and muscle tension with the help of a special machine.

Biopsy (BY-op-see): The removal of cells or tissues for examination by a pathologist. He or she may study the tissue under a microscope or perform other tests on the cells or tissue.

Brachytherapy (BRAY-kee-THAYR-uh-pee): A type of radiation therapy in which radioactive material sealed in needles, seeds, wires, or catheters is placed directly into or near a tumor. Also called implant radiation therapy, internal radiation therapy, and radiation brachytherapy.

Clinical stage: The stage of cancer that is based on all of the available information obtained before a surgery to remove the tumor.

Cryosurgery (KRY-o-SER-juh-ree): A procedure in which tissue is frozen to destroy abnormal cells. Liquid nitrogen is used to freeze the tissue. Also called cryoablation and cryosurgical ablation.

CT scan: A series of detailed pictures of areas inside the body taken from different angles. The pictures are created by a computer linked to an x-ray machine. Also called CAT scan, computed tomography scan, computerized axial tomography scan, and computerized tomography.

Diagnosis (DY-ug-NOH-sis): The process of identifying a disease, such as cancer, from its signs and symptoms.

Digital rectal examination (DRE): An examination in which a doctor inserts a lubricated, gloved finger into the rectum to feel for abnormalities.

Ejaculation (i-JAK-yoo-LAY-shun): The release of semen through the penis during orgasm.

Erectile dysfunction (ED) (ih-REK-tile dis-FUNK-shun): Not being able to have an erection of the penis adequate for sex. Also called impotence.

External beam radiation (RAY-dee-AY-shun): A type of radiation therapy that uses a machine to aim high-energy rays at the cancer from outside the body. Also called external radiation.

Gleason score (GLEE-sun): A system of grading prostate cancer tissue based on how it looks under a microscope. Gleason scores range from 2 to 10 and indicate how likely it is that a tumor will spread. A low Gleason score means that the cancer tissue is similar to normal prostate tissue and less likely to spread. A high Gleason score means that the cancer tissue is very different from normal prostate tissue and is more likely to spread.

Hormone therapy: Treatment that adds, blocks, or removes hormones. To slow or stop the growth of certain cancers (such as prostate and breast cancer), synthetic hormones or other drugs may be given to block the body's natural hormones. Sometimes surgery is needed to remove the gland that makes a certain hormone.

Incontinence (in-KAHN-tih-nens): Inability to control the flow of urine from the bladder (urinary incontinence) or the escape of stool from the rectum (fecal incontinence).

Intensity-modulated radiation therapy (IMRT) (in-TEN-sih-tee-MAH-juh-LAY-tid RAY-dee-AY-shun THAYR-uh-pee): A type of 3-dimensional radiation therapy that uses computer-generated images to show the size and shape of the tumor. Thin beams of radiation of different intensities are aimed at the tumor from many angles. This type of radiation therapy reduces the damage to healthy tissue near the tumor.

Laparoscopic prostatectomy (LA-puh-ruh-SKAH-pik PROS-tuh-TEK-toh-mee): Surgery to remove all or part of the prostate with the aid of a laparoscope (a thin, lighted tube attached to a camera).

Lobe: A portion of an organ, such as the prostate.

Lymph node (limf): A rounded mass of lymphatic tissue that is surrounded by a capsule of connective tissue. Lymph nodes filter lymph (lymphatic fluid), and store lymphocytes (white blood cells). They are located along lymphatic vessels. Also called a lymph gland.

MRI: A procedure in which radio waves and a powerful magnet linked to a computer are used to create detailed pictures of areas inside the body. These pictures can show the difference between normal and diseased tissue.

Medical oncologist (MEH-dih-kul on-KAH-loh-jist): A doctor who specializes in diagnosing and treating cancer usi ng chemotherapy, hormone therapy, biological therapy, and targeted therapy. A medical oncologist often is the main health care provider for someone who has cancer. A medical oncologist also gives supportive care and may coordinate treatment given by other specialists.

Medicated urethral system for erection (MUSE): A small pellet is inserted into the urethra using an applicator to help with erections.

Milliliter (MIH-luh-LEE-ter): A measure of volume in the metric system. One thousand milliliters equal one liter. Also called cc, cubic centimeter, and ml.

Nanogram: A measure of weight. One nanogram weighs a billion times less than one gram, and almost a trillion times less than a pound.

Nerve-sparing surgery: A type of surgery that attempts to save the nerves near the tissues being removed.

Osteoporosis (OS-tee-oh-puh-ROH-sis): A condition that is marked by a decrease in bone mass and density, causing bones to become fragile.

Pathological stage (PA-thuh-LAH-jih-kul stayj): The stage of cancer that is determined based on how the cells in the samples look under a microscope.

Pathology report (puh-THAH-loh-jee): The description of cells and tissues made by a pathologist based on microscopic evidence, and sometimes used to make a diagnosis of a disease.

Pelvis: The lower part of the abdomen, located between the hip bones.

Perineal prostatectomy (PAYR-uh-NEE-ul PROS-tuh-TEK-toh-mee): Surgery to remove the prostate through an incision made between the scrotum and the anus.

Prostate (PROS-tayt): A gland in the male reproductive system. The prostate surrounds the part of the urethra (the tube that empties the bladder) just below the bladder and makes a fluid that forms part of the semen.

Prostate cancer: Cancer that forms in tissues of the prostate (a gland in the male reproductive system found below the bladder and in front of the rectum).

Prostate-specific antigen (PSA)(PROS-tayt-speh-SIH-fik AN-tih-jen) : A protein made by the prostate gland and found in the blood. Prostate-specific antigen blood levels may be higher than normal in men who have prostate cancer, benign prostatic hyperplasia (BPH), or infection or inflammation of the prostate gland.

Prostate-specific antigen (PSA) test: A blood test that measures the level of prostate-specific antigen (PSA), a substance made by the prostate and some other tissues in the body. Increased levels of PSA may be a sign of prostate cancer.

Prostatectomy (PROS-tuh-TEK-toh-mee): Surgery to remove all or part of the prostate. Radical (or total) prostatectomy is the removal of the entire prostate and some of the tissue around it.

Radiation Oncologist (RAY-dee-AY-shun on-KAH-loh-jist): A doctor who specializes in using radiation to treat cancer.

Radiation therapy (RAY-dee-AY-shun THAYR-uh-pee): The use of high-energy radiation from x-rays, gamma rays, neutrons, and other sources to kill cancer cells and shrink tumors. Radiation may come from a machine outside the body (external beam radiation therapy). Or, it may come from radioactive material placed in the body near cancer cells (internal radiation therapy or brachytherapy).

Rectum: The last several inches of the large intestine closest to the anus.

Reproductive system (REE-proh-DUK-tiv SIS-tem): The organs involved in producing offspring. In men, it includes the prostate, the testes, and the penis.

Retropubic prostatectomy (re-tro-PYOO-bik pros-ta-TEK-toemee): Surgery to remove the prostate through an incision made in the wall of the abdomen.

Scrotum: In males, the external sac that contains the testicles.

Seminal vesicle (SEH-mih-nul VEH-sih-kul): A gland that helps make semen.

Standard therapy: Treatment that experts agree is appropriate, accepted, and widely used.

Testosterone (tes-TOS-teh-RONE): A hormone made mainly in the testes (part of the male reproductive system). It is needed to develop and maintain male sex characteristics, such as facial hair, deep voice, and muscle growth.

Tumor: An abnormal mass of tissue that results when cells divide more than they should or do not die when they should. Tumors may be benign (not cancer) or malignant (cancer). Also called neoplasm.

Urologist (yoo-RAH-loh-jist): A doctor who specializes in diseases of the urinary organs in females and the urinary and sex organs in males.

Watchful waiting (WACH-ful WAY-ting): Closely monitoring a patient's condition but not giving treatment unless symptoms appear or change. It is used in conditions that progress slowly, are hard to diagnose, or may get better without treatment.